Manel BOUDOKHANE
Olfa SAIDANE
Hiba BETTAIEB

Ankle involvement in adult juvenile idiopathic arthritis

Manel BOUDOKHANE
Olfa SAIDANE
Hiba BETTAIEB

Ankle involvement in adult juvenile idiopathic arthritis

Contribution of osteoarticular ultrasound of the ankle

ScienciaScripts

Imprint
Any brand names and product names mentioned in this book are subject to trademark, brand or patent protection and are trademarks or registered trademarks of their respective holders. The use of brand names, product names, common names, trade names, product descriptions etc. even without a particular marking in this work is in no way to be construed to mean that such names may be regarded as unrestricted in respect of trademark and brand protection legislation and could thus be used by anyone.

Cover image: www.ingimage.com

This book is a translation from the original published under ISBN 978-620-6-72592-3.

Publisher:
Sciencia Scripts
is a trademark of
Dodo Books Indian Ocean Ltd. and OmniScriptum S.R.L publishing group

120 High Road, East Finchley, London, N2 9ED, United Kingdom
Str. Armeneasca 28/1, office 1, Chisinau MD-2012, Republic of Moldova, Europe
Printed at: see last page
ISBN: 978-620-8-22172-0

Contents

LIST OF ABBREVIATIONS

JIA: Juvenile Idiopathic Arthritis

CRP: C-reactive protein

DAS 28: Disease activity score

EGP: Global assessment by the patient

VAS: Visual Analogue Scale

VAS dl: Visual analogue pain scale

EULAR: European League Against Rheumatism

HAQ: Health Assessment Questionnaire

ILAR: International League of Associations for Rheumatology

BMI: Body Mass Index

MRI: Magnetic Resonance Imaging

Mg: milligrams

Mg/l: milligrams per litre

Mm/h1: millimetre in the first hour

NAD: Number of painful joints

NAT: Number of swollen joints

RA: Rheumatoid arthritis

RM: Morning stiffness

RN: Night awakenings

VS: Sedimentation rate

INTRODUCTION

Juvenile idiopathic arthritis (JIA) is the leading cause of chronic inflammatory rheumatism in children [1-3]. Its incidence is estimated at between 0.8 and 22.6 per 100,000 children under the age of 16, and its prevalence is estimated at between 7 and 401 per 100,000 children [4].

According to the International League of Associations for Rheumatology (ILAR), it is defined as arthritis with no apparent cause, beginning before the age of 16, persisting for at least six months and comprising at least six different forms defined by clinical and biological inclusion and exclusion criteria (appendix 1) [5-7].

The polyarticular form is one of the most severe forms of JIA, which can lead to significant disability. [8]. This disability is partly due to joint damage in the feet [[9-10].

Damage to the talocrural joint is part of damage to the hindfoot. It is often unrecognised and can develop insidiously. However, it seems to be particularly affected, with an estimated prevalence of between 40% and 78% in the literature [[11,12].

In order to explore the involvement of the talocrural joint in juvenile idiopathic arthritis, we conducted a cross-sectional study in the rheumatology department of the Charles Nicolle Hospital with the following objectives:

- To assess ankle involvement in adult polyarticular JIA by clinical radiographic and ultrasound examination.

METHODS

1. Characteristics of the study

This was a single-centre cross-sectional study including all patients with polyarticular juvenile idiopathic arthritis (JIA) seen in adulthood, over a period of 18 months. Data collection was based on interviews with patients and their medical records archived in the Rheumatology Department of the Charles Nicolle Hospital.

2. Patients

2.1 Inclusion criteria

We included in our study patients with seropositive or seronegative polyarticular juvenile idiopathic arthritis (JIA) meeting the revised ILAR criteria (Edmonton 2004) [Appendix 1] aged 18 years and over.

2.2 Non-inclusion criteria

We did not include :

-Other forms of juvenile idiopathic arthritis (oligoarticular, enthesitic, arthritis with psoriasis, systemic and unclassified forms).

-Patients with congenital malformations of the feet.

2.3 Exclusion criteria

Excluded from the study:

-Patients whose files contained incomplete data preventing statistical analysis.

-Patients with comprehension problems.

3. Methods

3.1. Data collection

-Data was collected in the same way, by a single examiner (a rheumatology resident), using an information sheet drawn up in advance during a face-to-face interview with the patient.

- We then drew up a framework (Appendix 2) which included :

3.1.1 Socio-demographic data

-The sociodemographic data obtained from patient interviews included age, sex, geographical origin, professional status, marital status and level of education.

3.1.2 Clinical examination data

-We calculated the body mass index (BMI) for all our patients.

3.1.3 Parameters of juvenile idiopathic arthritis

3.1.3.1 Clinical parameters

- ❖ Patient's age at diagnosis.
- ❖ Duration of the evolution of JIA.
- ❖ How the disease is revealed.
- ❖ JIA activity parameters :
  - ➢ Number of painful joints (NAD) out of the 28 joints recommended by EULAR for calculating the DAS28 score [13].
  - ➢ Number of swollen joints (NAT).
  - ➢ Assessment of pain on a visual analogue scale (VAS) ranging from 0: no pain to 100: worst possible pain.

- Global evaluation of the disease by the patient (EGP).
- Duration of morning stiffness in minutes (MR).
- The number of night-time awakenings (NR).
- Calculation of disease activity score 28 (DAS28): this is a composite index of RA activity, calculated using the following formula: DAS28= [0.56 x √ (number of painful joints)] + [0.28 x √ (number of synovitis)] + [0.7 x Ln (VS or CRP)] + [0.014 x EGP] [1].

3.1.3.2 Biological parameters

-All patients underwent an inflammatory work-up including measurement of the sedimentation rate (ESR) in mm and C-reactive protein (CRP) in mg/ml.

3.1.3.3 Radiological data In our study, we took X-rays of the ankles, knees and pelvis to look for lower-limb involvement.

3.1.4 Parameters of talocrural damage

3.1.4.1 Functional signs

In our study, we looked for :

-The date of onset of talocrural damage.

-The delay between the onset of JIA and the onset of damage to the talocrural joint, and the different ways in which it may be revealed: pain, difficulty walking.

- Assessment of pain on a visual analogue scale (VAS) ranging from 0: no pain to 100: worst possible pain.

3.1.4.2 Clinical signs

- Pain or limitation was sought by passive mobilisation in flexion and extension of both ankles in our patients.

- Physical examination for synovitis.

3.1.4.3 Imaging signs

- **Radiological:** X-rays of the ankles in front and in profile were taken in our patients. Involvement of the talocrural joint was suspected in the presence of joint pinching, erosions or geodes, or even ankylosis. The radiographs were interpreted by a single rheumatologist.

- **Ultrasound:** osteoarticular ultrasound of the talocrural joints was performed by a single operator (rheumatologist) on an Esaote Mylab Gamma machine in all patients.

The presence of joint pinching, erosions, or cold or active synovitis of the talocrural joint was sought. We also looked for tendon involvement such as tenosynovitis of the fibular tendons or posterior tibial tendon.

3.2 Statistical analysis

- All data were entered using Statistical Package for Social Sciences (SPSS) version 23 for Windows.

3.2.1 Descriptive study

The descriptive study included :

- For qualitative variables, the calculation of absolute frequencies and relative frequencies (percentages).

- For quantitative variables, calculation of means, medians and standard deviations (standard derivations) with determination of extreme values (minimum and maximum).

3.2.2 Analytical study

- We divided our collated JIA patients into two groups as follows:

❖ **Group 1 (talocrural joint involvement+)**: Patients with talocrural joint involvement at diagnosis or during the course of JIA.

❖ **Group 2 (talocrural joint involvement)**: Patients who have not developed talocrural joint involvement.

- The analytical study was based essentially on a comparison of these two groups.

3.2.2.1 Comparison of averages

- Comparisons of 2 means were made using the non-parametric Mann-Whitney test (suitable for small numbers).

3.2.2.2 Comparison of percentages

Percentage comparisons were made using Fisher's two-tailed exact test (suitable for small numbers).

-In all statistical tests, the significance level (p) was set at 0.05.

4. Bibliographic research

- The bibliographic search was carried out in the electronic databases of Pub Med, Science direct and Cochrane to select articles of interest using the following key words: "juvenile idiopathic arthritis, talocrural joint", as well as their corollaries in English.

5. Conflicts of interest

- We declare no conflict of interest in relation to this work.

- All patients gave their oral consent to take part in the study.

RESULTS

DESCRIPTIVE STUDY

1. Characteristics of our population

1.1 Socio-demographic data

1.1.1 Frequency

- We enrolled 29 patients with polyarticular juvenile idiopathic arthritis during the study period.

1.1.2 Breakdown by gender

- The distribution of patients by sex is summarised in Figure 1, with a predominance of females, with a sex ratio of 0.16 (Figure 1).

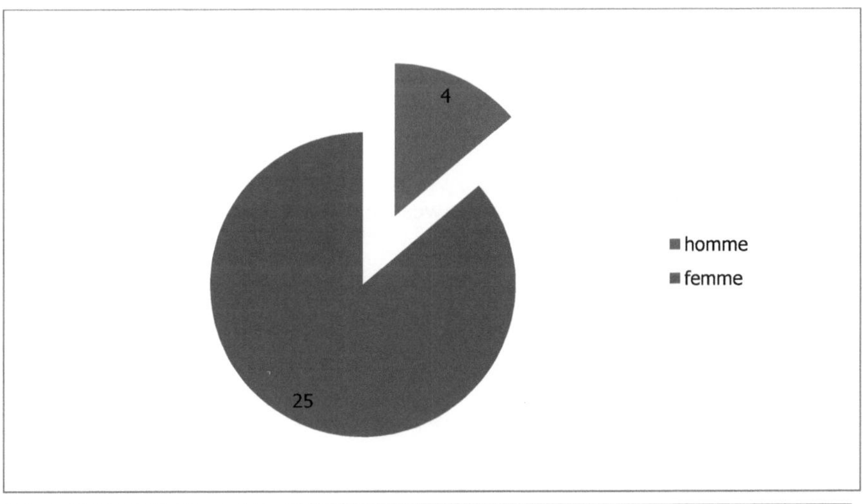

Figure 1. Breakdown of our patients by sex

1.1.3 Breakdown by age

- Our study population had an average age of 42.13 ± 12.51 years, ranging from a minimum age of 18 years to a maximum age of 65 years. The distribution of patients by age is summarised in Figure 2.

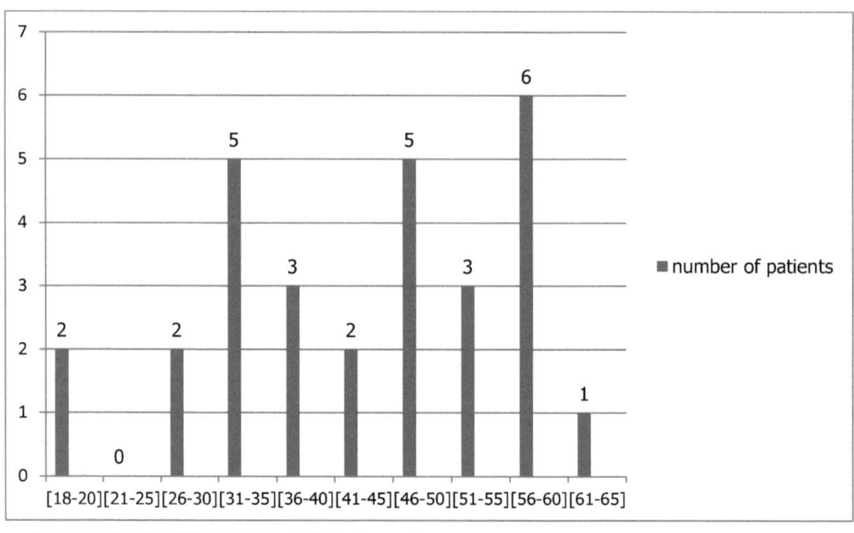

Figure2. Breakdown of patients by age group

1.1.4 Breakdown by geographical origin

- Most patients were from the north-west (62%) (Figure 3).

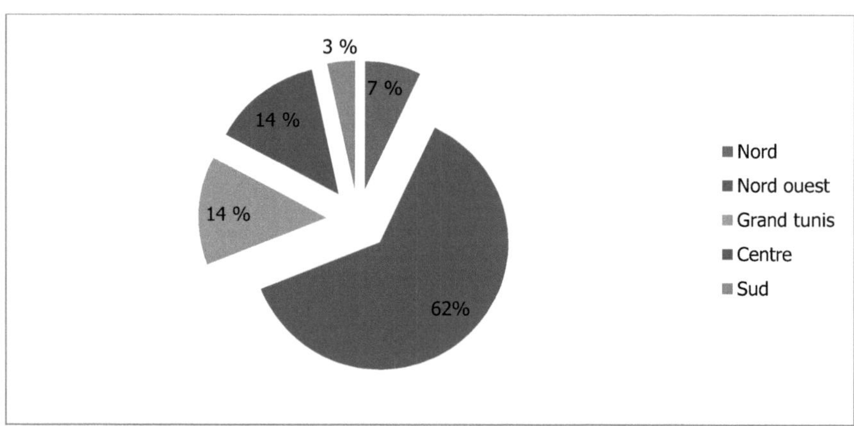

Figure 3. Breakdown of patients by geographical origin

1.1.5 Breakdown by level of education

- The majority of our patients had a primary education (Figure 4).

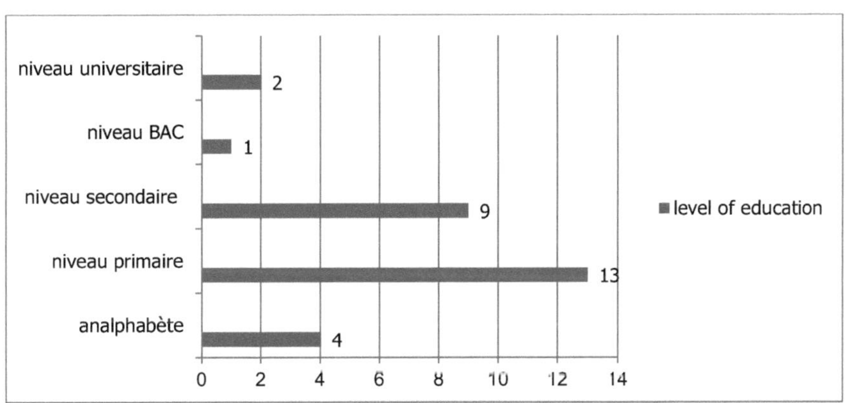

Figure 4. Distribution of patients by level of education

1.1.6 Breakdown by professional status

- Sixty-five per cent of our patients were unemployed, and in a large proportion of cases they attributed their unemployment to their illness-related disability (Figure 5).

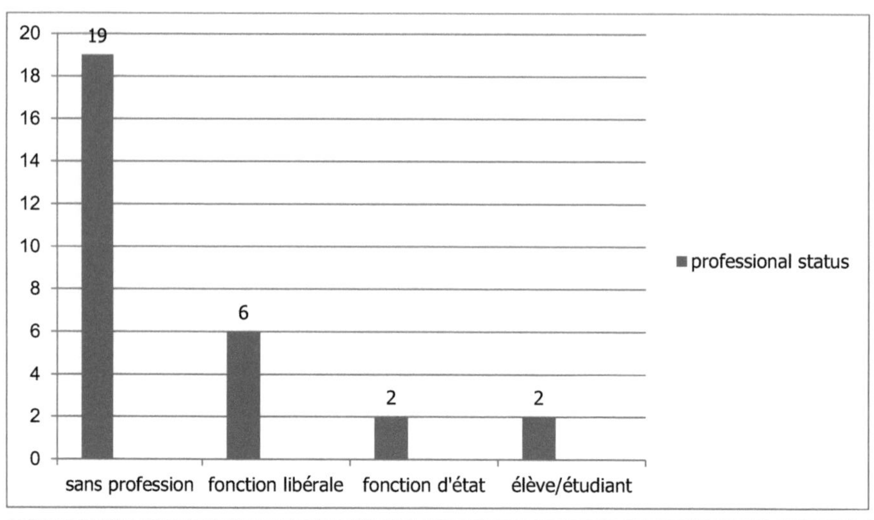

Figure 5. Breakdown of patients by professional status

1.1.7 Breakdown of patients by marital status

- Our patients were single in 48% of cases. The other patients were married (42%), divorced (7%) and widowed (3%).
- Among married, divorced and widowed patients, 28% had primary infertility.

1.1.8 Distribution of patients by body mass index (BMI).

- In our population, 51.7% of patients were overweight or obese (Figure 6).

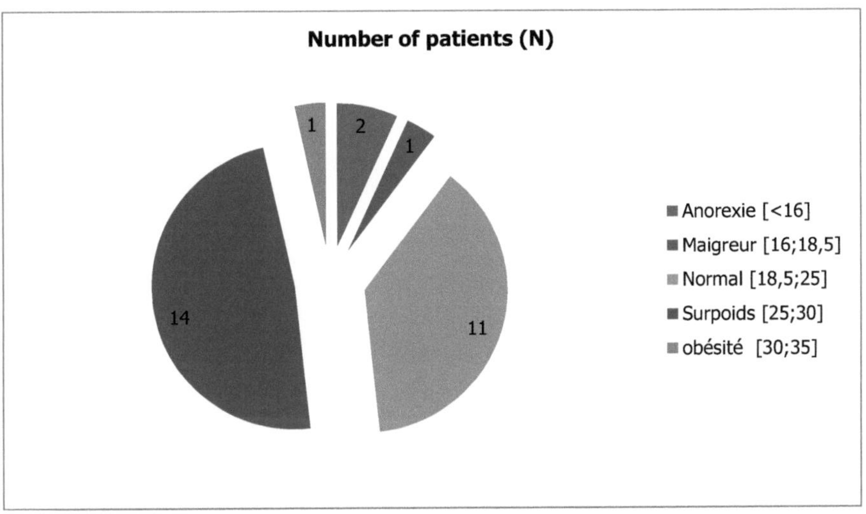

Figure 6. Distribution of patients according to BMI

1.2 Parameters of juvenile idiopathic arthritis (JIA)

1.2.1 Age at diagnosis of rheumatism

- The mean age at diagnosis of JIA was 11.24 ± 4.12 years, with extremes of 3 and 15 years.

1.2.2 How JIA is revealed

- Polyarthritis was the mode of onset of the disease in the majority of cases (52%) (Figure 7).

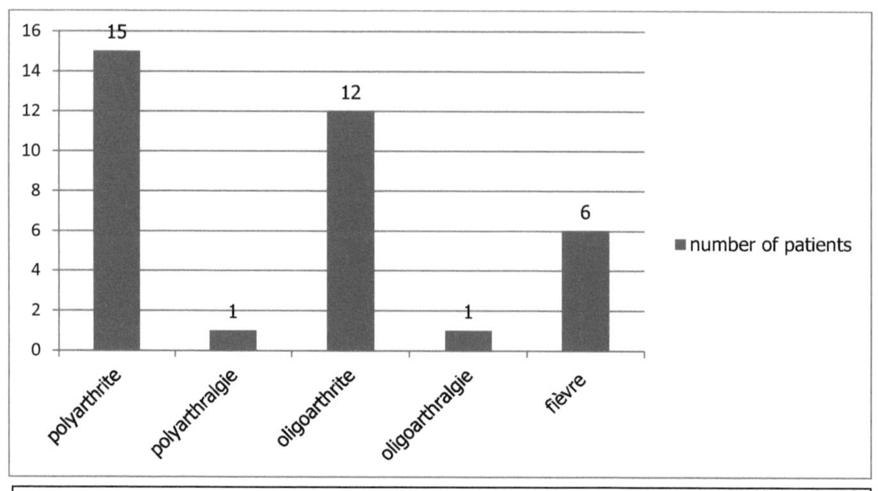

Figure 7. Distribution of patients according to the mode of onset of JIA

1.2.3 AJI activity parameters

- The various parameters of disease activity are summarised in Table I. Sixty-two per cent of patients had high disease activity, with a mean DAS28 VS score of 5.16±1.3 (Table I).

Table I: Parameters of JIA activity

parameters	median	Extreme
Duration of morning stiffness in minutes	60	[0-360]
Number of night-time awakenings	2	[0-4]
EVA pain	70	[0-100]
NAD	6	[0-28]
NAT	2	[0-14]
DAS 28 VS	5.3	[2,1-7,9]
DAS 28 CRP	4.5	[0,9-7,5]

NAD=number of painful joints, NAT=number of swollen joints, VAS pain=Visual Analogue Pain Scale.

1.2.4 Biological parameters of JIA

- Seventy percent of patients had a biological inflammatory syndrome (elevated SV and/or CRP) (Table II).

Table II: Biological parameters of JIA

Biological ignition parameter	median	extreme
VS (mm/h1)	40	[6-87]
CRP (mg/l)	14	[0,2-90]

VS=sedimentation rate, CRP=C-reactive protein

1.2.5 Radiological data

- Standard X-rays revealed :Involvement of the knees in 14 patients (48%).

- Coxitis in 10 patients (34%).

2. Characteristics of damage to the talocrural joint

- Of our patients, 23 (79%) had talocrural joint involvement diagnosed on standard radiographs and/or osteoarticular ultrasound.

2.1 Functional signs

2.1.1 The average time between foot involvement and onset of the disease

- The average delay between the onset of foot disease and the onset of the disease was 11.13 years, with a minimum of 0 years and a maximum of 48 years.

- The mean duration of foot disease was 21.17 ±16.66 years, with a minimum of one year and a maximum of 56 years.

2.1.2Revealing mode

- Involvement of the foot was revealed by various complaints, the most frequent of which was difficulty walking (Figure 8).

- The mean pain VAS was 69.31 ±34.53.

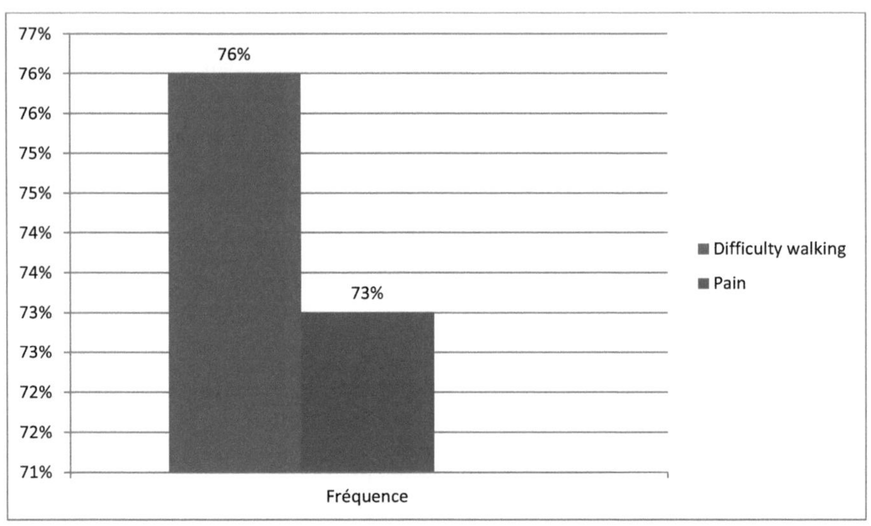

Figure 8. Distribution of patients by mode of onset of foot disease

2.2 Clinical signs

- Ankle instability was observed in 12 patients (41%).

- Ankle swelling was noted in 8 patients (28%).

- Mobility of the talocrural joint (flexion, extension) was limited and painful in 28% and 62% of cases respectively (Figure 9).

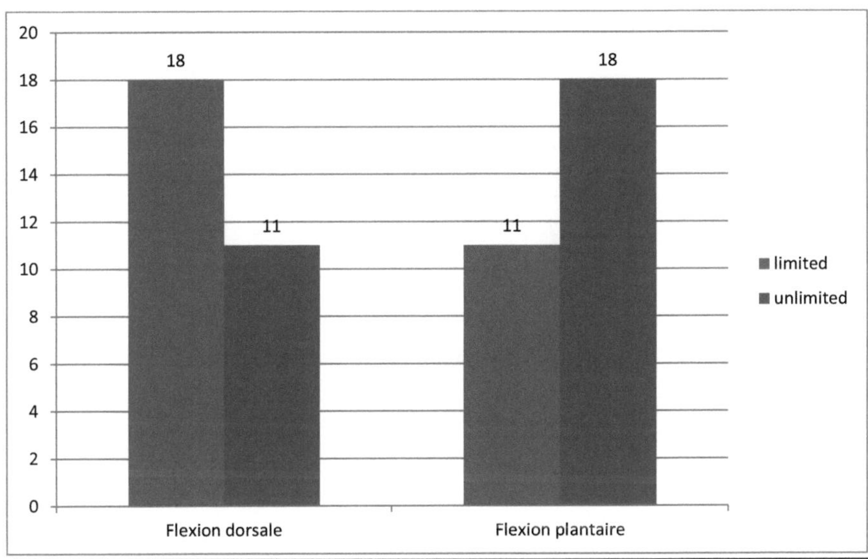

Figure 9. Distribution of patients according to talocrural joint mobility

2.3 Imaging signs

- On standard radiographs, the talocrural joint was abnormal in 16 patients (55%). We observed :

❖ talocrural pinch in 55% of cases.

❖ erosions and geodes in 21% and 10% of cases respectively.

- On ankle ultrasound, talocrural involvement was common: 72% (Table III).

Table III: The frequency of different abnormalities of the talocrural joint revealed by osteoarticular ultrasonography

Frequency (%)	Right	Left
Joint pinching	59 %	55 %
Cortical irregularity	17 %	10 %
Inactive synovitis	7 %	7 %
Active Synovitis	3 %	0 %

3. Assessment of fibular and posterior tibial tendon damage

- In our population, tenosynovitis of the fibular and/or posterior tibial tendons was noted in 11 patients (38%) on ultrasound (Figure 10).

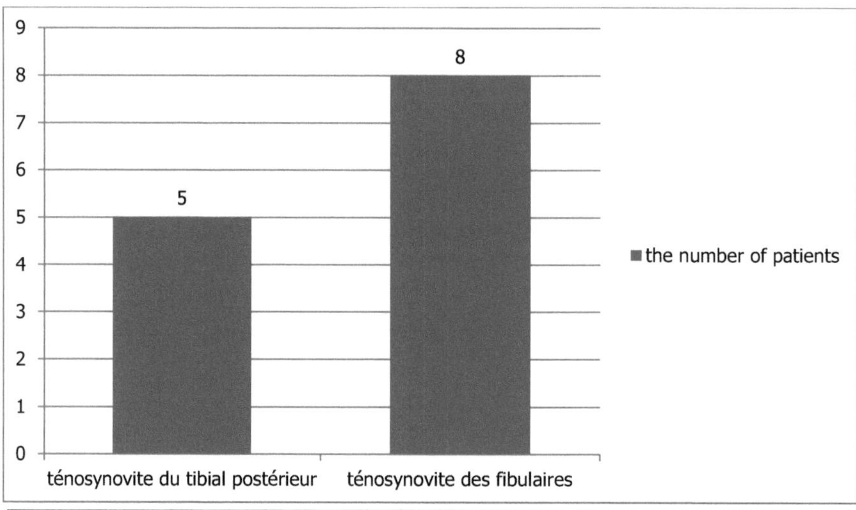

Figure 10. Frequency of fibular and posterior tibial tenosynovitis in our population

ANALYTICAL STUDY

1. **Comparison of socio-demographic parameters according to the presence or absence of damage to the talocrural joint**

- The various socio-demographic parameters did not appear to influence talocrural joint damage (Table IV).

Table IV: Comparison of socio-demographic parameters according to the presence or absence of damage to the talocrural joint

	Group1	Group 2	P
Age (average)	43.9± 12	39±13	0.39
Gender (female)	19	6	0.55
Education (N illiterate)	0	4	0.54
Employment status (N not working)	17	2	0.19
Marital status (N married)	10	3	0.65
Smoking(N)	5	0	0.55

N= number of patients, p= level of statistical significance, Group1= talocrural damage +, Group2= talocrural damage -.

-In our study, we found a statistically significant relationship between BMI and talocrural damage ($p=0.03$) (Figure 11).

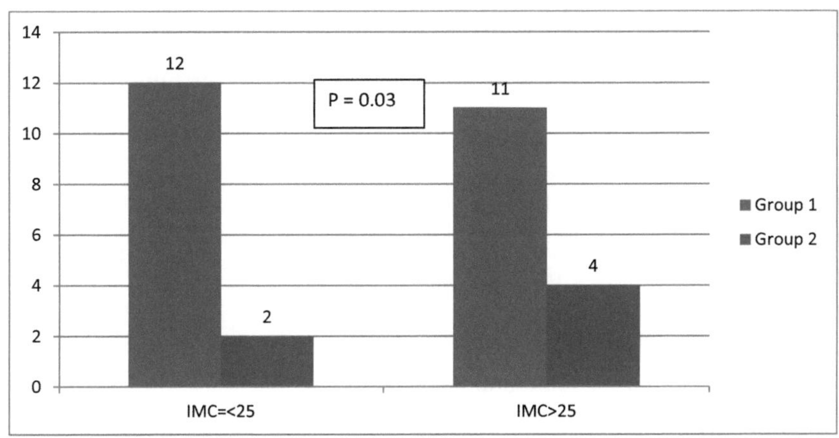

p= level of statistical significance, Group1= talocrural damage +, Group2= talocrural damage -.

Figure 11. Association between BMI and talocrural damage

2. Parameters related to juvenile idiopathic arthritis (JIA)

2.1. Clinical parameters

2.1.1. Start mode

- The onset of talocrural joint involvement was not influenced by the mode of onset of JIA. (Table V)

Table V: Comparison of the different ways in which JIA is revealed according to the presence or absence of damage to the talocrural joint

Revealing mode	Group 1 (N=)	Group 2 (N=)	P
Polyarthritis	11	4	0.65
Polyarthralgia	1	0	1
Oligoarthralgia	1	0	1
Oligoarthritis	10	2	1
Fever	6	0	0.29

N=number of patients, p=level of statistical significance, Group 1= talocrural damage +, Group 2= talocrural damage -.

2.1.2. Development time

- The duration of JIA was not significantly associated with the onset of talocrural involvement (p=0.68) (Table VI).

Table VI: Association between length of JIA course and talocrural involvement

	Group 1	Group 2	P
Length of time JIA has progressed (average/years)	11.39	10.17	0.68

p= level of significance, Group 1= talocrural damage +, Group 2= talocrural damage -.

2.1.3. Juvenile idiopathic arthritis activity parameters

- There was no statistically significant association between NAD, NAT and damage to the talocrural joint.

- We also found no association between the other parameters of JIA activity and the occurrence of talocrural joint damage (Table VII).

Table VII: Comparison of JIA activity parameters between the two groups

	NAD	NAT	EGP	EVAdl	SAR 28 vs	DAS 28crp	RM (min)		RN	HAQ
Group1 (M)	8,5	3,26	70,8	70,4	5,27	4,68	73		1,8	1,74
Group2 (M)	7,8	5,8	50	50	4,75	4,01	75		1,5	1,67
P	0,57	0,43	0,27	0,39	0,49	0,49	0,95		0,95	0,28

NAD=number of painful joints, NAT=number of swollen joints, EGP=global assessment by the patient, RM=morning stiffness, RN=night-time awakenings, VASdl=visual analogue pain scale, HAQ=functional index, p=level of significance, M=mean. Group 1= talocrural damage +, Group 2= talocrural damage -.

2.1.4. Biological parameters

- We found a statistically significant difference between the two groups in the presence of elevated CRP (Table VIII).

Table VIII: Relationship between the biological inflammatory syndrome and the occurrence of damage to the talocrural joint

The average	Group 1	Group 2	P
VS (mm/h1)	40,3±24,2	29,5±18,2	0,35
CRP (mg/l)	20,3±19,2	5,8±4.1	0, 02

SV=sedimentation rate, CRP=C-reactive protein, p=level of significance, Group 1=Talocrural +, Group 2=Talocrural-.

2.1.5. Radiological data

- There was a statistically significant association between knee and ankle involvement (Figure 12).

- We found no statistically significant difference between the two groups in terms of hip involvement.

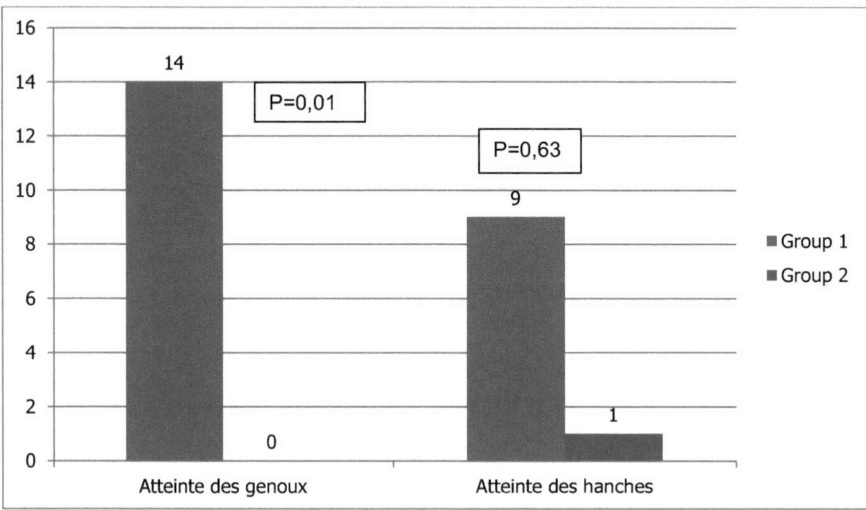

Group 1= talocrural damage +, Group 2= talocrural damage-, p=level of significance.

Figure 12. Relationship between the various joint injuries and talocrural damage

2.2. Relationship between fibular and posterior tibial tenosynovitis and talocrural damage

- Comparison of the two groups with regard to the presence of fibular and posterior tibial tenosynovitis revealed no statistically significant difference between the two JIA groups with or without talocrural involvement (Figure 13).

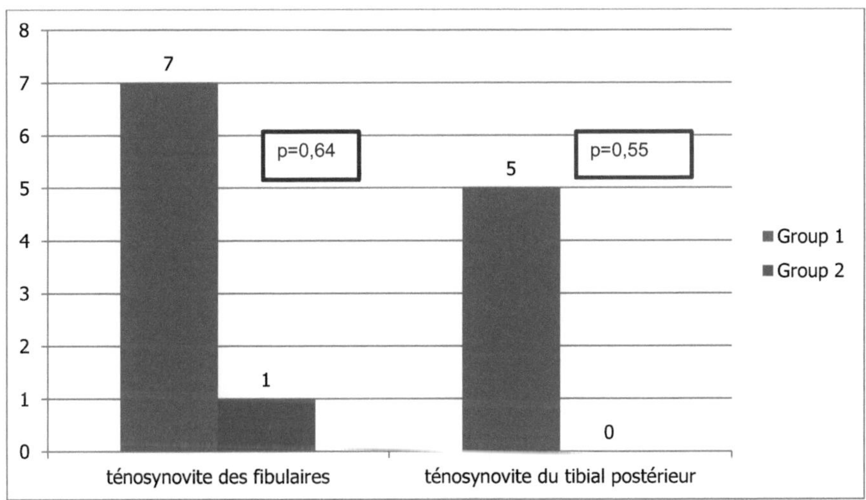

Group 1= talocrural damage +, Group 2= talocrural damage-, p=level of significance.

Figure 13. Relationship between the presence of tenosynovitis of the feet and damage to the talocrural bone

DISCUSSION

- **The main results of our study :**

- In our study, the occurrence of talocrural involvement during polyarticular juvenile idiopathic arthritis seen in adulthood was not negligible: 79% of our patients had talocrural joint involvement (23/29 patients).
- The average delay between the onset of foot disease and the onset of the disease was 11.13 years, with a minimum of 0 years and a maximum of 48 years.
- The mean duration of foot disease was 21.17 ±16.66 years, with a minimum of one year and a maximum of 56 years.
- Involvement of the foot was revealed by various complaints, the most frequent of which was difficulty walking: pain on walking requiring rest.
- Passive mobilisation of the talocrural joint by flexion and extension movements was limited and painful in 28% and 62% of cases respectively.
- Among the 23 patients with talocrural involvement, front and side X-rays of the ankles revealed talocrural involvement in 55% of cases.
- On ultrasound, involvement of the talocrural joint was frequent (72%).

✓ **The comparative study** showed that :

- BMI was significantly associated with the occurrence of talocrural damage (p=0.03).
- Patients with talocrural joint involvement had significantly higher CRP levels than the group without talocrural joint involvement (p=0.02).
- Talocrural involvement was significantly associated with knee involvement (p=0.01), while there was no statistically significant relationship with hip involvement.

- **The strengths of our study :**

1) The overall approach to damage to the talocrural joint, which is often underestimated and mislabelled in JIA, has not been the subject of enough studies. To our knowledge, this is the first nationwide study.

2) Our work included an interesting analytical study comparing two groups of JIA (with and without talocrural joint involvement), to determine the characteristics of talocrural joint involvement.

3) In addition to the clinical examination and standard radiological work-up, exploration of the talocrural joint included osteoarticular ultrasound.

- **Limitations of our study :**

Nevertheless, our study had some shortcomings:

1) The size of our JIA population was too small to provide statistically reliable results.

2) The duration of progression and monitoring of JIA was not identical for all patients, leading to heterogeneity in our study population.

- **Strengths of literature studies :**

1) In some studies, exploration of the talocrural joint included a clinical examination, radiography and osteoarticular ultrasound of the feet, or even MRI.

2) Some studies were prospective, which enabled a better assessment of the evolution of foot involvement in chronic inflammatory rheumatism.

3) The population size of some studies was large.

- **Weaknesses in literature studies :**

1) In the literature, there were few studies of talocrural involvement in JIA.

2) The majority of studies looked at JIA in children rather than adults.

1. Factors associated with talocrural damage in JIA

1.1 Socio-demographic parameters

❖ **Age**

- In our study, there was no association between age and talocrural involvement (p=0.39). This result is consistent with the study by Yano *et al.* which was carried out on a population of RA patients and showed that there was no statistically significant relationship between foot involvement and age (p=0.98). [9].

❖ **sex**

- In the literature, the female sex was a predictive factor of structural evolutivity [14]. In our study, 66% of patients with talocrural joint involvement were female, with no significant difference between the sexes (p=0.55).
- Similarly, the Spraul *et al.* study of JIA patients showed that there was no significant association between foot involvement and gender. [15].

❖ **BMI**

- In our study, we found a statistically significant relationship between BMI and talocrural damage (p=0.03).
- In a study conducted by Borman *et al.* on patients with RA, foot pain was significantly associated with BMI [16].

- Finally, in the literature, by analogy with JIA, a Japanese study of 5637 patients with RA found a significantly higher BMI in patients with foot involvement (p=0.004). [9].

1.2 AJI-related parameters

❖ Duration of development of JIA

- The average time between the onset of foot involvement and the onset of JIA varied in the literature. In chronic inflammatory rheumatic diseases, foot involvement was rarely inaugural. However, its frequency increased with the duration of the disease, reaching 50 to 90% depending on the series [[10, 17-19].

- In line with the literature, our study showed a delay in onset of foot involvement of 11.1 years [0; 48 years] from the onset of JIA.

❖ Revealing mode

- In our study, foot involvement was revealed in the majority of cases by walking difficulties. Similar results were found in rheumatoid arthritis, another chronic inflammatory rheumatic disease affecting the feet, where involvement of the feet and ankle interfered with walking in 75% of cases, i.e. 4 times more often than the hip and knee. [20].

❖ AJI activity parameters

- In a study of ankle involvement in RA, a significant association was found between ankle destruction and disease activity. [21].

- Furthermore, a study conducted by Rojas *et al.* on subjects with RA confirmed that the frequency of foot involvement increased with disease activity. [22].

- In the Japanese study of 5637 patients with rheumatoid arthritis, DAS 28 was significantly higher in the group of patients with foot involvement than in the group without foot involvement ($p<0.01$). [9]

❖ **Biological parameters**

- In our study, we found a statistically significant difference between the two groups with and without talocrural damage in the presence or absence of a biological inflammatory syndrome (CRP levels).

- In RA, the study by Yano *et al.* found higher values of SV and CRP ($p<10^{-3}$) in patients with foot involvement than in those without, which is consistent with our results. [9].

❖ **Radiological parameters**

- In our study, X-ray data confirmed the presence of destruction of the knees (48.3%) and hips (34.5%). We found a statistically significant association between knee and talocrural damage ($p=0.01$).

- In the Belt *et al.* study of RA patients, the ankles were more affected in patients with the most severe destruction. [[23].

2. Involvement of the talocrural joint in JIA

- On ultrasonography, involvement of the talocrural joint was observed in 21 patients (72%).

- In a Danish study of 30 children with JIA who met the ILAR criteria, talocrural involvement was detected ultrasonographically in 78% of cases [12].

- This could be explained by the greater sensitivity of ultrasound in the exploration of the hands and feet. [24].

- Similarly, several other studies have shown the superiority of ultrasound in detecting subclinical synovitis in the ankles and feet [25,26].

3. Tenosynovial involvement

- In our population, tenosynovitis of the fibular and/or posterior tibial tendons was noted on ultrasound in 11 patients (38%).
- In the literature, tenosynovitis was common in chronic inflammatory rheumatism [27, 28-30].
- In RA, Bouysset *et al.* found tenosynovitis on MRI in 81% of cases. This tenosynovitis was frequently associated with involvement of the hindfoot [27].
- Contrary to the literature, our study did not reveal a statistically significant association between the two groups of JIA with and without talocrural involvement.

CONCLUSIONS

Juvenile idiopathic arthritis (JIA) is the leading cause of chronic inflammatory rheumatism in children. For a long time, JIA was considered a childhood disease that died out in adulthood. However, in recent years it has been shown that it can remain active even into adulthood.

Few studies have been carried out on foot involvement in JIA. However, this joint location is common and has a significant impact on patients' function and quality of life.

Damage to the talocrural joint is part of damage to the hindfoot. It is often unrecognised and can develop insidiously.

In this single-centre, cross-sectional study of 29 patients with polyarticular JIA seen in adulthood and collected in the rheumatology department of the Charles Nicolle Hospital in Tunis over a period of 18 months, we proposed the following:

- To use clinical examination, radiography and osteoarticular ultrasound to assess ankle involvement in adult polyarticular JIA.

We did not include :

- Other forms of juvenile idiopathic arthritis (oligoarticular, enthesitic, arthritis with psoriasis, systemic and unclassified forms).
- Patients with congenital malformations of the feet

Two groups were compared:

- ❖ **Group 1 (talocrural joint involvement+)**: Patients with talocrural joint involvement at diagnosis or during the course of JIA.
- ❖ **Group 2 (talocrural joint involvement-)**: Patients who have not developed talocrural joint involvement+.

The clinical, paraclinical and evolutionary characteristics of JIA were collected and compared between the two groups.

Various socio-demographic and clinical data (number of painful joints, number of swollen joints, joint mobility) were recorded.

The results of biological (VS, CRP) and radiological examinations were recorded, as well as JIA activity parameters (DAS28 score). All parameters were entered into an SPSS file.

The study population consisted of 25 women and 4 men (sex ratio 0.16) with an average age of 42.1 ± 12.5 years.

The majority of our patients had a primary education (13/29, or 45%).

Sixty-five per cent of our patients were unemployed, and a large proportion of them attributed their unemployment to an illness-related disability.

Our patients were single in 48% of cases. The remaining patients were married (42%), divorced (7%) and widowed (3%). Among married, divorced and widowed patients, 28% had primary infertility.

In our population, 51.7% of patients were overweight or obese.

The mean age of onset of JIA was 11.2 ± 4.12 years, with a mean duration of rheumatic disease of 31.7 ± 14 years. Polyarthritis precipitated JIA in 52% of cases.

On examination, the median number of painful and swollen joints was 6 (0-28) and 2 (0-14) respectively. The mean DAS28 VS score was 5.1 ± 1.3.

The median SV was 40 mm/h1 (6-87). The median CRP was 14 mg/l (0.2-90). Seventy per cent of patients had a biological inflammatory syndrome (elevated SV and/or CRP).

In our population, radiographs showed knee and hip involvement in 14 (48%) and 10 (34%) patients respectively.

Talocrural involvement was observed in 79% of our patients who had polyarticular juvenile idiopathic arthritis in adulthood.

The mean time to onset of foot disease was 11.1 years (0-48 years). The mean duration of foot disease was 21.1 ±16.6 years (1-56 years). Foot disease was revealed by various complaints, the most frequent of which was difficulty walking.

Passive mobilisation of the talocrural joint by flexion and extension movements was limited and painful in 28% and 62% of cases respectively.

Of the 23 patients with talocrural involvement, foot X-rays showed this in 55% of cases.

On ultrasonography, involvement of the talocrural joint was observed in 21 patients (72%). The presence of tenosynovitis of the fibular and posterior tibial joints was not significantly related in the two JIA groups.

According to the analytical study, BMI was significantly associated with the occurrence of talocrural damage ($p=0.03$), which is consistent with the results of the literature.

Patients with talocrural joint involvement had significantly higher CRP levels than those without ($p=0.02$).

There was a statistically significant association between damage to the talocrural joint and damage to the knees ($p=0.01$).

In the light of our results and the data in the literature, we propose the following recommendations:

- ✓ Improve doctors' awareness of the need to screen for talocrural damage in JIA.
- ✓ Early and frequent use of osteoarticular ultrasound to explore the talocrural joint.

Prospective studies on a larger scale are essential to enable a better assessment of damage to the talocrural joint in JIA and to improve patient management.

REFERENCES

1. Crayne CB, Beukelman T. Juvenile idiopathic arthritis: oligoarthritis and polyarthritis. Pediatr Clin North Am. 2018;65(4):657-74.

2. Dannecker GE, Quartier P. Juvenile idiopathic arthritis: classification, clinical presentation and current treatments. Horm Res. 2009;72 (Suppl) 1:4-12.

3. Batu ED. Glucocorticoid treatment in juvenile idiopathic arthritis. Rheumatol Int. 2018.doi: 10.1007/s00296-018-4168-0.

4. Manners PJ, Bower C. Worldwide prevalence of juvenile arthritis why does it vary so much? J Rheumatol. 2002;29(7):1520-30.

5. Petty RE, Southwood TR, Manners P, Baum J, Glass DN, Goldenberg J, et al. International League of Associations for Rheumatology classification of juvenile idiopathic arthritis: second revision, Edmonton, 2001. J Rheumatol. 2004;31(2):390-2.

6. Foeldvari I, Bidde M. Validation of the proposed ILAR classification criteria for juvenile idiopathic arthritis. International League of Associations for Rheumatology. J Rheumatol. 2000;27(4):1069-72.

7. Ravelli A, Martini A. Juvenile idiopathic arthritis. Lancet. 2007;369(9563):767-78.

8. 10. Ringold S, Weiss PF, Beukelman T, DeWitt EM, Ilowite NT, Kimura Y, et al. 2013 Update of the 2011 American College of Rheumatology Recommendations for the Treatment of Juvenile Idiopathic Arthritis: Recommendations for the Medical Therapy of Children With Systemic Juvenile Idiopathic Arthritis and Tuberculosis Screening Among Children Receiving Biologic Medications. Arthritis Rheum. 2013;65(10):2499-512.

9. Yano K, Ikari K, Inoue E, Sakuma Y, Mochizuki T, Koenuma N, et al. Features of patients with rheumatoid arthritis whose debut joint is a foot or ankle joint: A 5,479-case study from the IORRA cohort. PLoS One. 2018;13(9):1-10.

10. van der Leeden M, Steultjens M, Dekker JH, Prins AP, Dekker J. The relationship of disease duration to foot function, pain and disability in rheumatoid arthritis patients with foot complaints. Clin Exp Rheumatol. 2007;25(2):275-80.

11. Katz PP, Morris A, Yelin EH. Prevalence and predictors of disability in valued life activities among individuals with rheumatoid arthritis. Ann Rheum Dis. 2006;65(6):763-9.

12. Laurell L, Court-Payen M, Nielsen S, Zak M, Boesen M, Fasth A (2011). Ultrasonography and color Doppler in juvenile idiopathic arthritis: diagnosis and follow-up of ultrasound-guided steroid injection in the ankle region. A descriptive interventional study. Pediatric Rheumatology, 9(1), 4.

13. van der Heijde DM, Jacobs JW. The original "DAS" and the "DAS28" are not interchangeable: comment on the articles by Prevoo et al. Arthritis Rheum. 1998;41(5):942-5.

14. Syversen SW, Gaarder PI, Goll GL, Odegard S, Haavardsholm EA, Mowinckel P, et al. High anti-cyclic citrullinated peptide levels and an algorithm of four variables predict radiographic progression in patients with rheumatoid arthritis: results from a 10-year longitudinal study. Ann Rheum Dis. 2008;67(2):212-7.

15. Spraul G, Koenning G. A descriptive study of foot problems in children with juvenile rheumatoid arthritis (JRA). Arthritis Care Res. 1994;7(3):144-50.

16. Borman P, Ayhan F, Tuncay F, Sahin M. Foot problems in a group of patients with rheumatoid arthritis: an unmet need for foot care. Open Rheumatol J. 2012;6:290-5.

17. McKinley JC, Shortt N, Arthur C, Gunner C, MacDonald D, Breusch SJ. Outcomes following pantalar arthrodesis in rheumatoid arthritis. Foot Ankle Int. 2011;32(7):681-5.

18. Scott DL, Smith C, Kingsley G. Joint damage and disability in rheumatoid arthritis: an updated systematic review. Clin Exp Rheumatol. 2003;21 (Suppl) 31:S20-7.

19. Goksel Karatepe A, Gunaydin R, Adibelli ZH, Kaya T, Duruoz E. Foot deformities in patients with rheumatoid arthritis: the relationship with foot functions. Int J Rheum Dis. 2010;13(2):158-63.

20. Thould AK, Simon G. Assessment of radiological changes in the hands and feet in rheumatoid arthritis. Their correlation with prognosis. Ann Rheum Dis. 1966;25(3):220-8.

21. Belt EA, Kaarela K, Maenpaa H, Kauppi MJ, Lehtinen JT, Lehto MU. Relationship of ankle joint involvement with subtalar destruction in patients with rheumatoid arthritis. A 20-year follow-up study. Joint Bone Spine. 2001;68(2):154-7.

22. Rojas-Villarraga A, Bayona J, Zuluaga N, Mejia S, Hincapie ME, Anaya JM. The impact of rheumatoid foot on disability in Colombian patients with rheumatoid arthritis. BMC Musculoskeletal Disord. 2009;10:67.

23. Belt EA, Kaarela K, Kauppi MJ. A 20-year follow-up study of subtalar changes in rheumatoid arthritis. Scand J Rheumatol. 1997;26(4):266-8.

24. Haslam KE, McCann LJ, Wyatt S, Wakefield RJ. The detection of subclinical synovitis by ultrasound in oligoarticular juvenile idiopathic arthritis: a pilot study. Rheumatology. 2010;49(1):123-7.

25. Inamo, J., Kaneko, Y., Sakata, K., & Takeuchi, T. Impact of subclinical synovitis in ankles and feet detected by ultrasonography in patients with rheumatoid arthritis. International Journal of Rheumatic Diseases. 2018.

26. Sant'Ana Petterle G, Natour J, Rodrigues da Luz K, et al. Usefulness of US to show subclinical joint abnormalities in asymptomatic feet of RA patients compared to healthy controls. Clin Exp Rheumatol 2013;31:904-912.

27. Bouysset M, Tavernier T, Tebib J, Noel E, Tillmann K, Bonnin M, et al. CT and MRI evaluation of tenosynovitis of the rheumatoid hindfoot. Clin Rheumatol. 1995;14(3):303-7.

28. Suzuki T, Okamoto A. Ultrasound examination of symptomatic ankles in shorter-duration rheumatoid arthritis patients often reveals tenosynovitis. Clin Exp Rheumatol. 2013;31(2):281-4.

29. Javadi S, Kan JH, Orth RC, DeGuzman M. Wrist and ankle MRI of patients with juvenile idiopathic arthritis: identification of unsuspected multicompartmental tenosynovitis and arthritis. AJR Am J Roentgenol. 2014;202(2):413-7.

30. Rooney ME, McAllister C, Burns JFT. Ankle disease in juvenile idiopathic arthritis: ultrasound findings in clinically swollen ankles. J Rheumatol. 2009;36(8):1725-9.

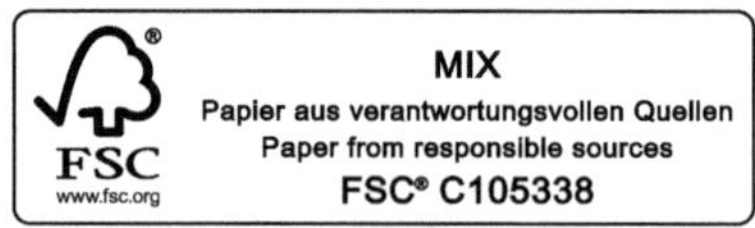

Printed by Books on Demand GmbH, Norderstedt / Germany